I0423892

FRUIT INFUSTED WATER:

Top 35 Vitamin Water Recipes For Fat Loss, Detox, And Better Health!

KATYA JOHANSSON

Copyright © 2016. All Rights Reserved.

Table of Contents

Introduction

It is SUPER essential to stay appropriately hydrated for the duration of the day, water is no joke! Being appropriately hydrated will give your body a chance to work taking care of business, you won't feel as drained or torpid and considerably appetite might be died down.

Be that as it may, such a large number of individuals don't drink enough water in the day! The prescribed water admission is 8 some water a day for a grown-up, and this will build the more physical action you finish. I have recently discharged my fresh out of the box new 1L drink bottle which is ideal for conveying in your exercise center or satchel, which makes it SO natural to recollect to stay hydrated!

In the event that you are one of those individuals that battles to drink water since it is exhausting, or you incline toward the essence of pop - I have the best formulas for you! These four natural product mixed water combos are the BEST.

Tips and Tricks

You can imbue water with any number of herbs, flavors, palatable blooms, leafy foods vegetables! Here are a few thoughts:

1. **Herbs**: Rosemary, thyme, mint, basil, cilantro, parsley

2. **Flavors**: Cinnamon sticks, cardamom cases, new ginger, cloves, vanilla bean

3. **Palatable blooms**: Rose, lavender, citrus blooms, hibiscus, pansies, and violets (or any that are 100% pesticide free)

4. **Natural product**: Berries (new or solidified), melon, tropical organic products, citrus, apples, pears

5. **Vegetables**: Fresh Cucumber, celery, fennel, carrots

6. **Water**: Filtered water is incredible, yet in the event that you don't have a filtration framework, faucet water is fine as well.

1. Amazing Naturally Flavored Water

Ingredients

- Strawberry Flavored Water:
- 4-6 strawberries, hulled and quartered
- ½ lemon, cut
- Little modest bunch of basil, scrunched
- Ice and frosty separated water
- Watermelon Flavored Water:
- 2 cuts of watermelon, cut into thirds or quarters
- Little modest bunch of basil, scrunched
- Ice and frosty separated water

Method

1. Fill your juice pitcher to the top with ice and organic product.
2. Marginally scrunch up the basil so it discharges its flavor. Spread with cool sifted water.
3. This water is ideal on the off chance that you give the water a chance to mix no less than 60 minutes. In case you're inpatient (like me), jab a couple openings in your organic product with a fork for moment flavor.

2. Healthy Blueberry Orange Water

Ingredients

- 6 glasses water
- 2 mandarin oranges, cut into wedges
- a modest bunch of blueberries
- ice

Method

1. Join all fixings in a pitcher and put in the refrigerator for 2-24 hours to permit the water to implant.
2. You can likewise crush in the juice of one mandarin orange and obfuscate the blueberries to increase season a bit.
3. Serve chilly.

3. Amazing Fruit Infused Water

Ingredients

- Natural product Infused Water Flavor Ideas
- Raspberry (or strawberry) lemon - any berry combined with lemon winds up with a light lemonade flavor!
- Watermelon mint - super reviving!
- Tropical (mango pineapple) - this one turns out sweeter than the others, however in an absolutely decent manner!
- citrus cucumber (lemon, lime, orange, cucumber)
- Different organic products to attempt: apples, honeydew, cantaloupe, blueberries, blackberries, peaches
- Attempt crisp herbs as well! Rosemary, basil, mint

Method

1. Add coveted organic products to a pitcher and afterward load with water. Permit organic product to splash for 2-8 hours in the cooler and afterward appreciate!
2. You can include as much or as meager natural product as you'd favor. Include more natural product for more flavor and sweetness for your waters.

4. Healthy Strawberry, Lime, Cucumber and Mint infused water

Ingredients

- 1 glass cut strawberries
- 1 glass cut cucumbers
- 2 limes, cut
- ¼ glass crisp mint takes off
- Ice blocks
- Water

Method

1. In a half-gallon jug, or a 2 quart pitcher, layer the strawberries, cucumbers, lime cuts, and mint leaves with the ice solid shapes.
2. Fill container or pitcher with water. Give chill for 10 minutes, and afterward a chance to appreciate!

5. Healthy Blueberry Lavender Water

Ingredients

- 1/2 half quart Blueberries
- Palatable Flowers (use Lavender Flowers) - to taste
- 64 ounces Water

Method

1. Add Fruits and palatable blooms to a pitcher of water.
2. Cover, and chill for no less than 30 minutes.
3. Strain, then include ice and fill tall glasses and serve.

6. Amazing Cantaloupe, Honey with Mint Agua Fresca

Ingredients

- ½ c water
- ½ c nectar
- 4 c (around 2 lbs) melon cut into 1 inch pieces
- ¼ c new lime juice (around 2 limes)
- 2 Tbsp new mint takes off
- ¼ tsp salt
- shining water or club pop
- mint sprigs for trimming

Method

1. Consolidate the nectar and water in a little pot and warmth over medium low warmth until water and nectar are joined and simply starting to bubble, around 2-4 minutes. Expel from warmth and cool somewhat.
2. Consolidate nectar syrup, melon, lime juice, mint leaves, and salt in a blender and puree until smooth.
3. Utilizing a fine coincided sifter or a bit of cheesecloth, strain the melon blend into another compartment. Dispose of solids. You ought to wind up with around 2 measures of fluid.
4. In every glass, pour ½ c of the melon juice over ice. Fill whatever is left of the glass with shimmering water or club pop and mix to blend. On the other hand, you can blend a balance of melon squeeze and shimmering water in a pitcher with ice and fill glasses as required. Trim with a mint sprig and appreciate!

7. Tasty Kiwi Cucumber Agua Fresca

Ingredients

- 6 kiwis, peeled
- 1 vast cucumber, peeled and seeded
- 4 parcels Splenda (or other no calorie sweetener)
- 6 glasses water, separated
- Additional kiwi cuts for topping

Method

1. Place the kiwi, cucumber, Splenda and some water in a blender and puree until smooth, around 3-4 minutes.
2. Exchange to a pitcher and blend in the remaining some water.
3. Serve chilled over ice. Trim with kiwi cuts

8. Delicious Honeydew and Raspberry Agua Fresca

Ingredients

- 1 (5 lb.) ready honeydew melon
- ½ glass preparing sugar (likewise called "superfine" or "ultrafine")
- 5 limes, squeezed
- 1 glass raspberries (for trimming)

Method

1. Sliced the melon down the middle, expel seeds with a spoon, then cut substance from peel and cut into lumps. Put half of the melon in a vast blender and procedure until melted. Empty the melted melon into a fine work sifter set over a huge dish.
2. Utilize a spatula to press the melon into the sifter, permitting the juice to crush through into the dish. Sometimes rub the substance off of the strainer to permit more squeeze to exchange to the dish. Rehash with remaining melon.
3. Exchange melon juice to a huge pitcher and include some water.
4. Consolidate lime squeeze and sugar in a little bowl, then mix until sugar is broken up. Empty the lime-sugar blend into the pitcher and mix well. Serve over ice, embellished with raspberries.

9. Healthy Watermelon Coconut Agua Fresca

Ingredients

- 1 (3 pound) seedless watermelon, cubed (around 5 mugs)
- 4 mugs (1 quart) coconut water
- 2 tablespoons crisply crushed lime juice (from 1 medium lime)

Method

1. Puree the watermelon in a blender. Place a fine-work strainer over a pitcher and precisely pour the pureed watermelon through the sifter. Dispose of mash.
2. Mix in coconut water and lime juice.
3. Chill, secured, until icy - no less than 60 minutes. Serve over ice.

10. Healthy Berry, Peach and Coconut

Ingredients

- 1 container natural blueberries
- 1 container natural blackberries
- 2 donut peaches, hollowed and cut into half-creep wedges
- 6 glasses spring or sifted water
- 2 glasses unsweetened natural coconut water
- 1 gallon clean glass jug with top

Method

1. Place blueberries and blackberries into the base of your jug, then the peach cuts on top.
2. Pour the spring water and coconut water into the jug. Blend the water, spread with a cover and place water into the icebox for no less than one hour or overnight for the best flavor. Drink inside two days.

11. Amazing Kiwi Cocktail

Ingredients

- 3-4 ready kiwis, peeled and meagerly cut (or smashed for more flavor)
- 2 quarts sifted or spring water

Method

1. Add the cut kiwis to a 64-ounce Mason jug or pitcher.
2. Include the sifted water.
3. Refrigerate until frosty and appreciate.

12. Healthy Strawberry, Basil and Cucumber

Ingredients

- 3 basil leaves generally slashed
- 1 strawberry cut
- 3-5 cuts of cucumber
- Ice
- Water

Method

1. Join every one of the fixings in a vast glass, and let sit for no less than 5 minutes before getting a charge out of.

13. Amazing Raspberry Lemon

Ingredients

- 2 glasses natural raspberries
- 8 glasses spring or sifted water
- 1 vast natural lemon, cut into half-crawl cuts
- 2 dried Medjool dates
- 1 gallon clean glass container with cover

Method

1. Place raspberries into the base of your container. Include the dates, then layer the lemon cuts on top. Empty water into container and spot top on top.
2. Place water into the fridge and let imbue for 60 minutes.

14. Tasty Mixed Melon

Ingredients

- 1 glass melon pieces
- 1 glass watermelon pieces
- 1 glass honeydew pieces
- 2 quarts sifted or spring water

Method

1. Add your melons to a 64-ounce Mason jug or pitcher.
2. Pour the water over top and chill. Serve over ice.

15. Delicious Orange, Strawberry and Mint

Ingredients

- 1/4 container new mint
- 1/2 container strawberries, cut
- 1/2 orange, cut
- 16 ounces separated water

Method

1. Put all products of the soil into the bricklayer container.
2. Fill to best with water.
3. Seal bricklayer jolt firmly and let it sit overnight in the fridge.

16. Amazing Pineapple Ginger

Ingredients

- 1 glass new pineapple pieces (pulverized for increasingly a sweeter taste)
- 1-inch piece ginger, daintily cut
- 2 quarts separated or spring water

Method

1. Add the pineapple and ginger to a 64-ounce Mason container or pitcher.
2. Pour the water over top and refrigerate until cool. Serve over ice.

17. Healthy Cucumber Lavender Mixer

Ingredients

- 1 cucumber, daintily cut
- 1 teaspoon dried culinary lavender, or 2 new lavender sprigs
- 2 quarts separated or spring water

Method

1. Add the cucumbers and lavender to a 64-ounce Mason container or pitcher.
2. Include the separated water. In the case of utilizing dried lavender, strain before serving.
3. Refrigerate until cool and appreciate.

18. Amazing Orange-Kiwi Infused Water

Ingredients

- some water or shimmering water
- 2 measures of ice
- 1 orange, cut
- 2 kiwis, peeled and cut

Method

1. Consolidate all in an expansive bricklayer jug or container and drink promptly or let sit in cooler for 1-4 hours to absorb extra flavor.

19. Cool Raspberry-Mint Infused Water

Ingredients

- some water or shimmering water
- 2 measures of ice
- 1 container raspberries, entirety
- modest bunch of mint

Method

1. Combine all in a huge artisan jug or container and drink promptly or let sit in ice chest for 1-4 hours to absorb extra flavor.

20. Healthy Blueberry-Lime Infused Water

Ingredients

- some water or shining water
- 2 measures of ice
- 1 container blueberries, entirety
- 1/2 limes, cut

Method

1. Combine all in a huge bricklayer container or container and drink promptly or let sit in ice chest for 1-4 hours to absorb extra flavor

20. Healthy Strawberry-Basil Infused Water

Ingredients

- some water or shining water
- 2 measures of ice
- 1 container strawberries, cut
- modest bunch basil

Method

1. Combine all in a huge bricklayer jug or container and drink quickly or let sit in cooler for 1-4 hours to absorb extra flavor

21. Amazing Lemon-Cucumber Infused Water

Ingredients

- some water or shimmering water
- 2 measures of ice
- 1 lemon, cut
- 10 dainty cuts of cucumber

Method

1. Combine all in a huge artisan container or container and drink quickly or let sit in ice chest for 1-4 hours to absorb extra flavor.

22. Unique Infused Water

Ingredients

- some water or shimmering water
- 2 measures of ice

Method

1. Combine each of the above elements for a super-fruity imbued water
2. Combine all in an expansive artisan jug or container and drink promptly or let sit in ice chest for 1-4 hours to absorb extra flavor.

23. Healthy Fruit mixed water

Ingredients

- 16 oz bricklayer container
- 1/2 container water
- 1/2 container natural product
- 1/4 container ice
- 2 mint leaves (discretionary)

Method

1. Place natural product in the base of your container. Pour water in and blend organic product around. Push on the natural product daintily with a spoon to discharge a portion of the flavors. Include mint leaves if fancied.
2. Refrigerate for no less than 60 minutes (can even do overnight). Include ice just before serving. Appreciate!

24. Amazing Citrus and Mint Infused Water

Ingredients

- 1 orange cut
- 1 lemon cut
- crisp mint clears out

Method

1. Fill a pitcher with water, include cuts of lemons and oranges and top with crisp mint from my herb garden.
2. Give it a chance to sit for 60 minutes in the ice chest before serving. Appreciate!

25. Delicious Alfalfa Arnold Palmer

Ingredients

- 1 section - lemon Juice
- 1 section - horse feed nectar syrup
- 1 section - water
- 2 sections - unsweetened tea

Method

For horse feed nectar syrup:
1. 2 sections Alfalfa nectar
2. 1 section HOT water
3. Consolidate fixings. Blend until disintegrated.

For beverage readiness:
1. Consolidate, blend. Refrigerate.
2. Serve over ice.

26. Amazing Agua de Limon

Ingredients

- Juice of 12 to 15 little limes
- 1 container - nectar
- 2 quarts - water
- Modest bunch - mint, discretionary

Method

1. Blend juice with nectar and water in pitcher until consolidated. Taste for sweetness and alter as needs be.

27. Delicious Spiced Honey Echinacea

Ingredients

- 4 - Echinacea tea bags
- 4 - cinnamon sticks
- 20 - entire cloves
- 1/2 container - nectar
- 1/4 container - crisp lemon juice

Method

1. Heat water to the point of boiling in a medium pan. Include tea sacks, cinnamon, and cloves ; let stew for 5 minutes.
2. Expel cinnamon and cloves and mix in nectar and lemon juice. Place in fridge until chilled (approx. 60 minutes). Pour over ice and enhancement with crisp lemon cuts. May substitute chamomile tea for the Echinacea tea.

28. Healthy Strawberry Lime Water

Ingredients

- strawberries (entire or cut),
- 2 limes (cut or quartered).

Method

1. In a half-gallon container, or a 2 quart pitcher, layer the strawberries and lime cuts with ice 3D shapes. Fill your jug or pitcher with water.
2. Give it a chance to marinate for around 10 minutes, and afterward appreciate!

29. Delicious Strawberry Cucumber Water

Ingredients

- 8 ounces strawberries
- 1/2 a cut cucumber

Method

1. Mix Strawberries and cucumber into a 2 quart pitcher of ice water. Refrigerate 2 to 4 hours to permit the fixings to implant.

30. Healthy Mango Ginger Water

Ingredients

- 1 inch Ginger Root, peeled and cut
- 1 container Frozen Mango-new is fine as well

Method

1. To peel the ginger utilize the back of a spoon or a vegetable peeler, simply peel the part that you will utilize.
2. Utilizing a sharp blade cut ginger into 3-4 coin measured cuts. You need them about the size and thickness of the coin.
3. Drop into your pitcher and include the mango.
4. Top with some ice and after that include with water
5. Place in your refrigerator for 1-3 hours before serving.
6. When serving include a couple solidified mango pieces in a lovely glass for ice 3D squares.

31. Delicious Lime Cucumber Mint Water

Ingredients

- 1 lime, daintily cut
- 5 inch cucumber, cut into rings
- 5 mint takes off
- 2 measures of ice
- Water

Method

1. In a huge pitcher, include the lime and cucumbers. Over the pitcher press and marginally contort the mint, don't tear separated you just need to tenderly discharge the oils, add the mint leaves to the pitcher. Top with ice and water. Give the pitcher a chance to sit in the ice chest for 1 hour before serving.
2. At the point when the water is down to 1/4 full in the pitcher, refill with water and place back in the ice chest. You can do this few times. Store in the cooler up to 24 hours.

32. Healthy Fruit Infused Water with Pears, Cranberries and Clementine

Ingredients

- 1 Pear meagerly cut
- 1 Clementine Orange cut into 8ths
- 1 tbsp. Dried Cranberries
- 1 tsp. All Spice Berries (look like pepper corns)

Method

1. Top w/1.5 mugs ice and afterward top off with water and let sit 3 hours in ice chest before drinking.
2. The key here is to cut your organic product as meagerly as you can with the goal that you get the most flavor. On the off chance that you need sweeter include an apple and another orange.

33. Delicious Tropical Pineapple and Orange Infused Water

Ingredients

- 1 orange, daintily cut
- 1/2 container pineapple, daintily cut
- 2 measures of ice
- Water

Method

1. Pineapple Orange Infused Water DetoxIn an extensive pitcher, include the orange and pineapple cuts. Top with ice and water. Give the pitcher a chance to sit in the cooler for 1 hour before serving.
2. At the point when the water is down to 1/4 full in the pitcher, refill with water and place back in the refrigerator. You can do this few times. Store Tropical Pineapple and Orange Infused Water in the ice chest up to 24 hours.

34. Amazing Mango Ginger Water

Ingredients

- 1 inch Ginger Root, peeled and cut
- 1 container Frozen Mango-new is fine as well

Method

1. To peel the ginger utilize the back of a spoon or a vegetable peeler, simply peel the part that you will utilize. Utilizing a sharp blade cut ginger into 3-4 coin estimated cuts. You need them about the size and thickness of the coin.
2. Drop into your pitcher and include the mango.
3. Top with some ice and after that include with water.(the ice is essential, it holds down the ginger and mango to mix the water)
4. Place in your cooler for 1-3 hours before serving.
5. When serving include a couple solidified mango pieces in a beautiful glass for ice 3D shapes.

35. Amazing Strawberry Lime Spritzer

Ingredients

- 8 Frozen or Fresh Strawberries
- 1 Lime
- 1-2 liters of Pellegrino or Club Soda-you can likewise utilize level water

Method

1. Cut the strawberries into three pieces and drop into the water or fill an implantation pitcher, then cut the lime into 10 wedges and add to the water.
2. Chill for 3-4 hours and serve, on the off chance that you like, have a go at making some strawberry and lime ice 3D shapes on the off chance that you are presenting with level water.
3. In an ice-3D square plate place one strawberry cut and a lime cut, spread with water and stop for 3-4 hours.

One Last Thing...

If you enjoyed this book or found it useful I'd be very grateful if you'd post a short review on Amazon.

Your support really does make a difference and I read all the reviews personally so I can get your feedback and make this book even better.
Thanks again for your support!

www.ingramcontent.com/pod-product-compliance
Lightning Source LLC
Chambersburg PA
CBHW061804280526
45787CB00003BA/1477

9781533189387